A PATIENT'S GUIDE TO

DENTAL IMPLANTS

ALL-ON-4 ®

First Printing: 2017

ISBN 978-1-947744-07-3

Twisted Key Publishing, LLC
405 Waltham Street
Suite 116
Lexington, MA 02421

www.twistedkeypublishing.com

Ordering Information: Special discounts are available on quantity purchases by corporations, associations, educators, and others. For details, contact the publisher at the above listed address.

US trade bookstores and wholesalers: Please contact Twisted Key Publishing, LLC by email twistedkeypublishing@gmail.com.

A PATIENT'S GUIDE TO

DENTAL IMPLANTS

ALL-ON-4 ®

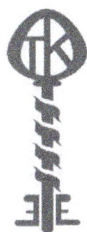

TWISTED KEY
publishing

2017

A Patient's Guide To Understanding All-On-4®

The decision to get dental implants is rarely quick or easy for most people. Few adults start life with a plan to replace all their teeth. It starts with a few cavities, a crown or two, a root canal, a bridge... Before they know it, thousands of dollars have been spent on procedure after procedure to try and save their teeth.

All-on-4® dental implants are a permanent solution to a full range of ongoing dental problems. This book is designed to give you a better idea of how the process works and what you can expect.

Meet Trevor

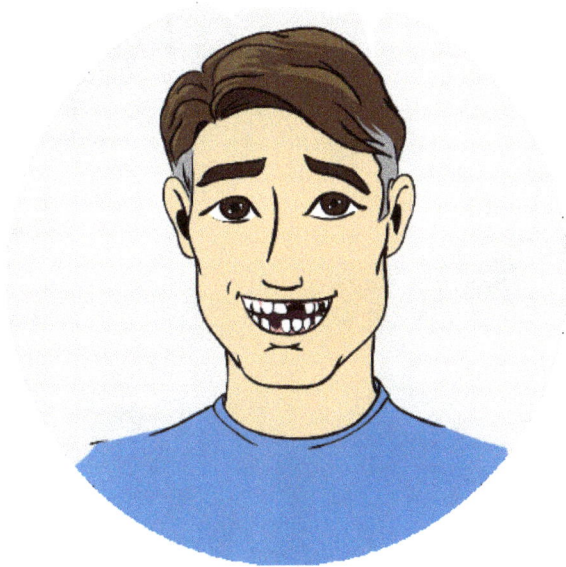

Trevor is our patient for today, and we'll be following him through the exciting journey of getting All-on-4® Dental Implants, allowing you to see what the experience is like before, the day of, and after the procedure.

Why All-on-4® Dental Implants?

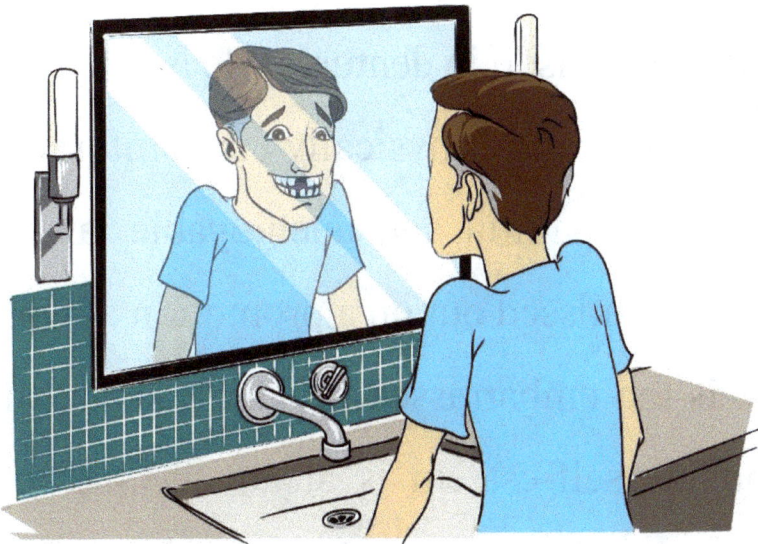

Trevor has been suffering for years with dental problems. He has had teeth pulled, crowns, and bridges, and now his dentist is suggesting dentures. Trevor is a teacher with an active lifestyle; he can't imagine himself in dentures. He is extremely frustrated and physically uncomfortable. Eating is painful and unenjoyable, and he recently missed out on a promotion at work. He is too embarrassed to have a social life, and his self-esteem is at an all-time low. After searching for a solution online, Trevor comes across dental implants and a procedure called All-on-4®. He decides to schedule an exam to find out if he is a candidate for the All-on-4® procedure.

The All-on-4® ends the cycle of repetitive and progressive dental procedures. It gives you a full, beautiful, natural-looking, and natural-feeling smile, restoring 90% of your natural bite force and eliminating painful dental issues.

First Visit – CT Scan

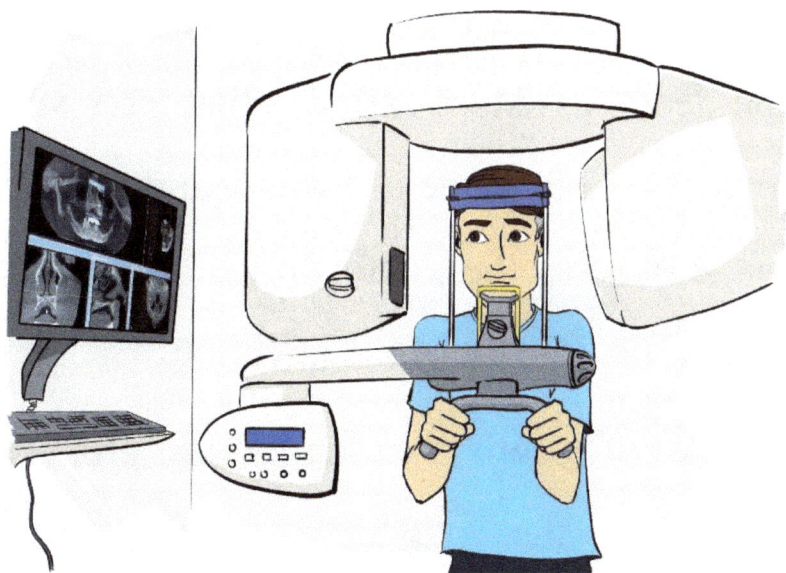

Trevor arrives at the office and meets with a friendly treatment coordinator. After the coordinator asks Trevor a few questions about his medical history, a dental assistant arrives to take a CT scan of Trevor's jaw. The dental assistant explains that a CT scan provides a 3D image of his jaw and that this image enables the doctor to see the height, width, and density of his jawbone.

A CT scan is essential for properly evaluating the patient's existing bone density. The CT scan is completely painless and takes about four minutes.

The Exam

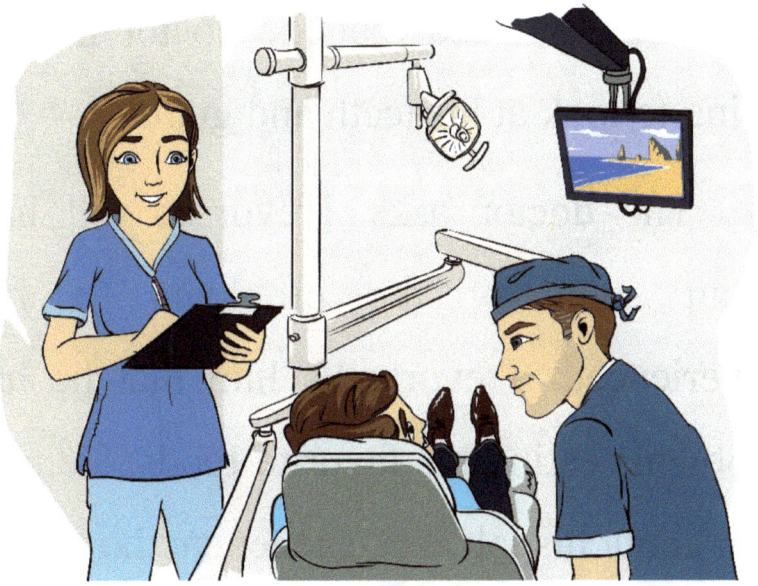

After the CT scan, Trevor is taken to an exam room. After years of painful exams, he is apprehensive. When the doctor enters the room, Trevor is assured that the exam will not be painful and that the doctor is only going to look at his teeth and gums.

The doctor asks Trevor to tell him about some of the problems he has experienced. Trevor tells him that he has problems eating his favorite foods. He tells him about his job as a teacher and how he is embarrassed to smile. He talks about trying his best to save his teeth, but now they have become loose and painful.

After their talk, the doctor reassures Trevor that he is a good candidate for the

All-on-4® and that they will review his CT scan and go over his options.

The exam is extremely gentle. The teeth and gums are examined, and a TMJ (temporomandibular joint) exam is performed – as is a head and neck cancer screening.

CT Review – 3D X-ray

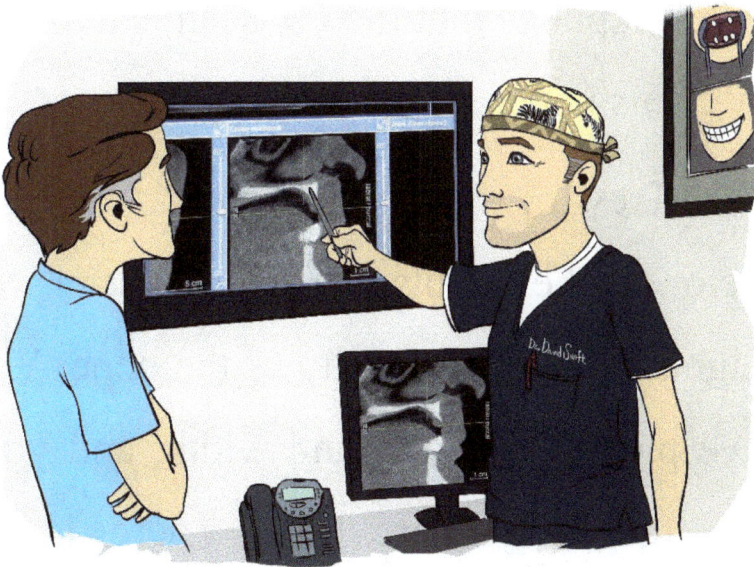

Trevor feels like he has finally found the answer! He begins to think about himself having a brand-new set of teeth. Up on the wall, a TV screen displays his CT scan. The doctor explains that the CT scan is a 3D X-ray of his upper and lower jawbones.

"Trevor, what I look for," says the doctor as he points to the CT scan, "is height, width, and density of the bone. You have plenty of height and width, and your bone quality is excellent. There is no practical solution available to save your remaining natural teeth. You are a perfect candidate for All-on-4®."

Trevor is filled with excitement. "When can I begin?!!"

The CT scan is extremely important because this 3D X-ray lets the doctor know if you have enough bone height and width for placement of implants. It also allows the doctor to see if there is any infection or other issues.

Impressions

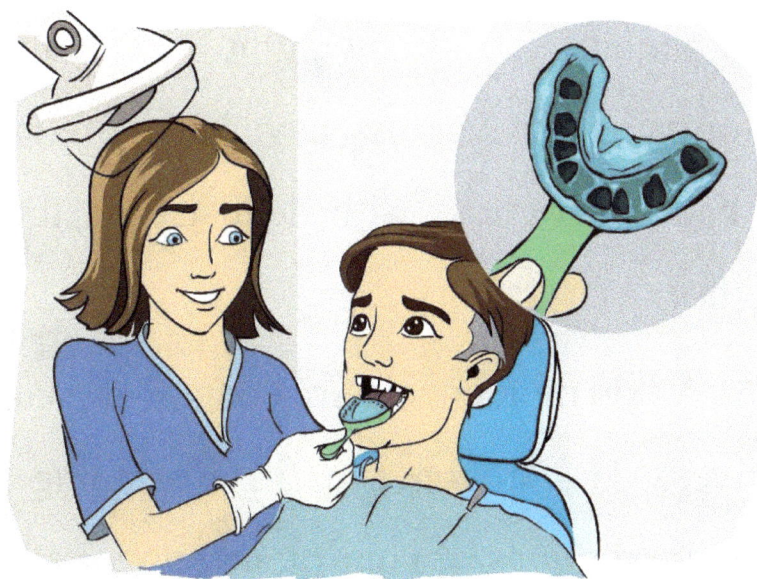

"We can get things started right away," the doctor tells Trevor. "I'll get a dental assistant and we'll take impressions."

The doctor shakes Trevor's hand and congratulates him, knowing how difficult it is for patients when they have had a lifetime of bad experiences with dentists and their teeth.

A few moments later, a dental assistant arrives. "Hi, Trevor, I'm Jill. I'm going to take impressions of your mouth, and the lab will use these impressions to help guide them as they create your new teeth."

Dental impressions can be either a mold or a digital scan. Once impressions are made, they are sent to a lab, where a lab technician will begin to make a brand-new set of custom teeth.

The Importance of Pictures

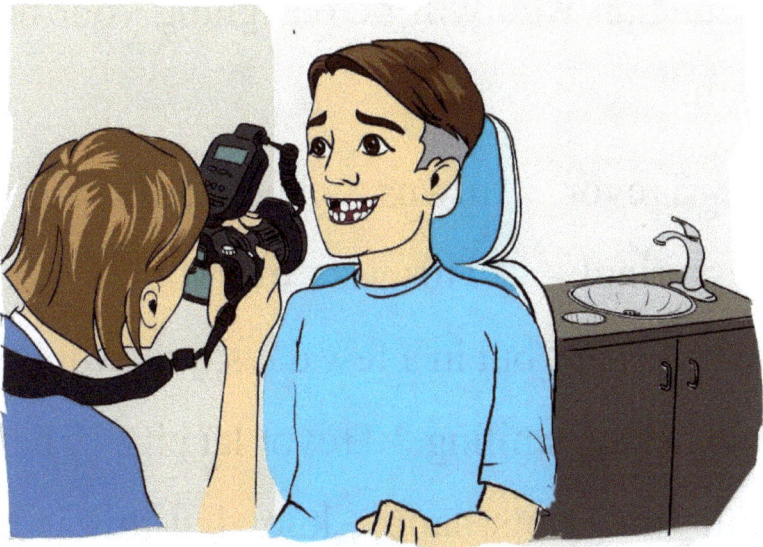

After finishing the impressions, Jill talks to the patient. "Trevor, I'm going to take some pictures of your smile and your face. These pictures will go to the lab technician who will be designing your new teeth."

Trevor frowns, but Jill smiles reassuringly. "This is everyone's least favorite part, but in a few days, you won't be able to stop smiling." Trevor laughs. "Thank you, Jill." He's happy, knowing this is the last photo he will take without a perfect smile.

Taking pictures is extremely important because it allows the lab technician to see the patient's personality, the shape of their face, and important things such as how much of their teeth or gums show when they smile. A fully custom set of teeth will be ready for the patient on the day of their surgery.

Surgery Day

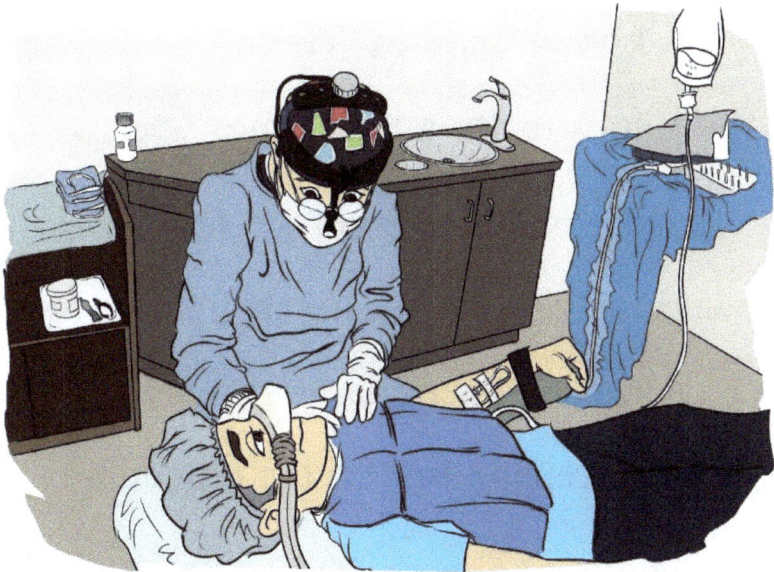

The day of Trevor's surgery arrives. Trevor is excited, but nervous as well. The doctor pats Trevor on the shoulder and smiles. "You're gonna be just fine."

"I know," smiles Trevor. "I've been waiting for this for a long time."

The doctor spends a few minutes answering Trevor's questions, helping to put him at ease. Then Trevor's sedation is started to prepare him for the procedure.

Sedation allows the patient to be relaxed and comfortable.

IV Sedation

IV sedation is considered moderate sedation because you are not completely asleep. IV sedation or Intravenous Conscious Sedation is administered via IV. IV sedation gives the doctor a high level of control over the effects and consistency of the sedation. Since IV sedation is delivered intravenously, the effects are felt very soon. Many dentists use IV sedation in conjunction with Nitrous Oxide, otherwise known as laughing gas, to help relieve any anxiety the patient may have about the procedure.

Most patients awaken after the procedure with little or no recollection that anything was done.

Placing the Implants

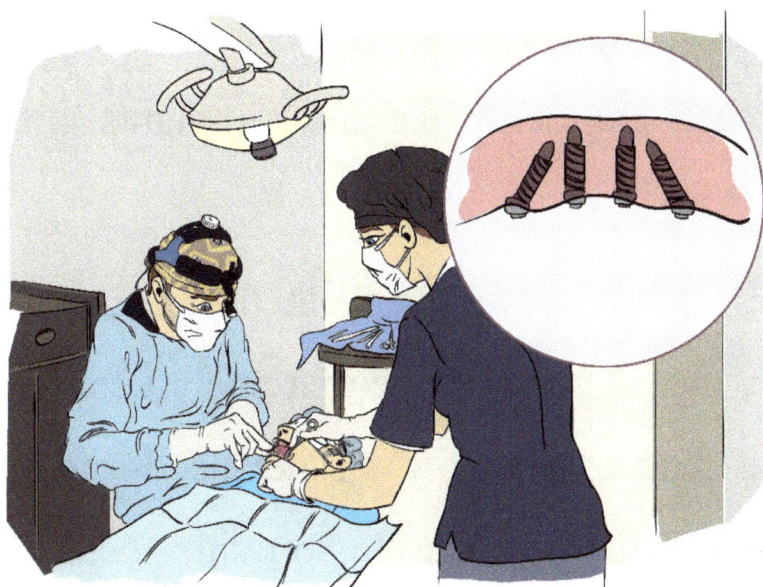

Once Trevor is comfortably sedated, the doctor gently removes Trevor's remaining teeth. Next, he places four titanium implants in the top jaw and tests each implant to make sure it is extremely secure. He then places four implants in the bottom jaw.

When removing teeth for the All-on-4®, the doctor must be extremely gentle, as the bone and soft tissue needs to be preserved in order to provide beautiful recipient sites for the new implants. The All-on-4® procedure is incredibly strong because two of the implants are at an angle, and two are arranged vertically, in each jaw.

The Dental Lab

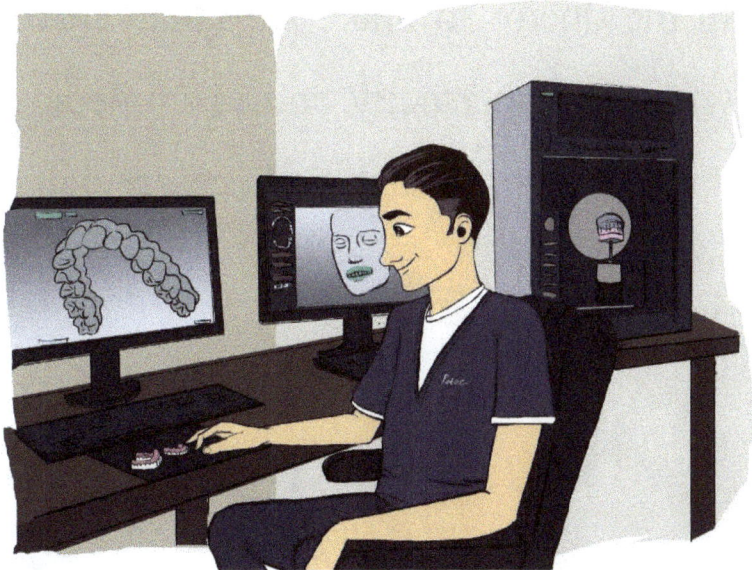

The dental lab has worked meticulously to create a beautiful set of teeth for Trevor. When the surgery is complete, the technician is there to work one-on-one with the doctor to make sure that Trevor's new teeth fit perfectly and to immediately make any changes that are necessary.

Trevor's New Teeth Are Ready

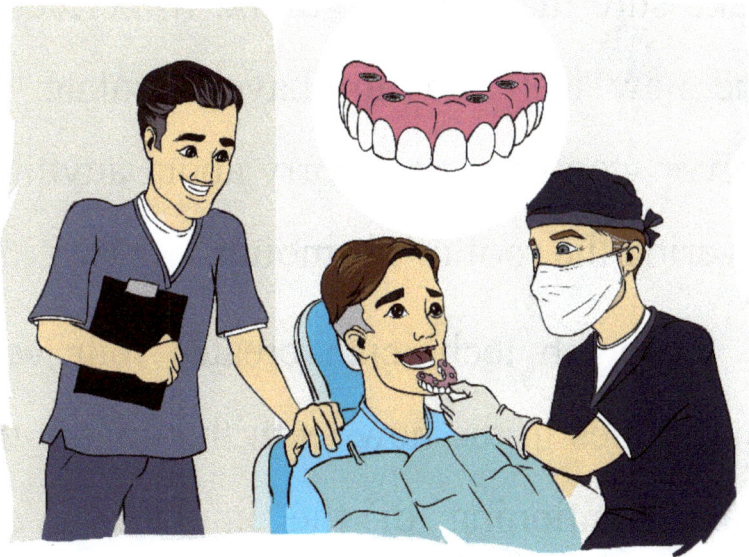

After the surgery, Trevor slowly awakes. The lab technician will begin aligning Trevor's new teeth to the implants. The lab technician will work diligently to make sure that they align and fit perfectly. The new teeth do not have a palate, so Trevor won't have to worry about anything covering the roof of his mouth.

The lab technician creates four very small holes in the new teeth that match the exact positioning of the implants. Very small screws will secure the new teeth in place. The new teeth will look completely natural and will return the patient's bite back to about 90% of the bite force they had when their original teeth were healthy and strong.

A Brand-New Smile

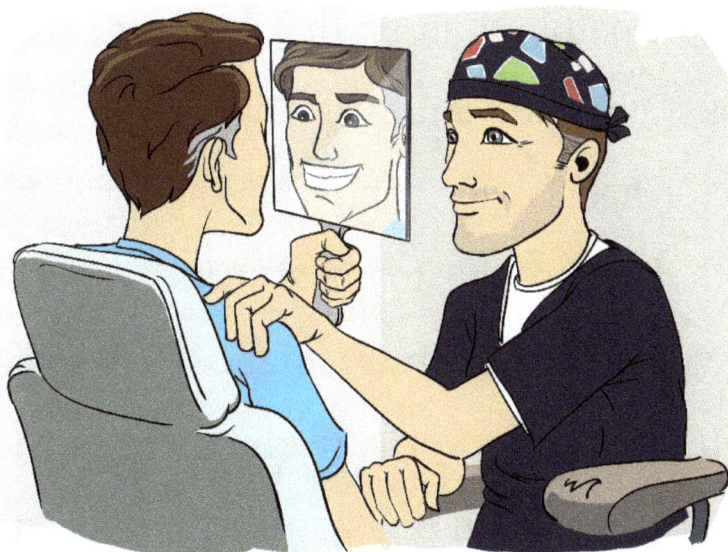

After adjusting the new teeth, the lab technician lets the doctor know that Trevor's teeth are ready!

"Trevor, you did great," says the doctor, patting him on the shoulder. Trevor looks up and smiles. "Thank you." The doctor has Trevor gently bite and grind his teeth. He does this to make sure that the bite is even and his teeth are aligned. After a few adjustments, Trevor is ready to see his new smile! "Are you ready to see your new teeth?" asks the doctor, smiling. He hands Trevor a mirror. Emotion fills Trevor's voice. "They are beautiful. Thank you." "You're welcome, Trevor. You were amazing."

Trevor stares into the mirror. He knows he will never have to be ashamed of his smile again. His new teeth look incredibly natural, and they feel like his own. This is Trevor's first set of teeth; in six months, he will get a second set. The doctor tells Trevor that there will be very little or no pain the next day and that most people only take an ibuprofen or two.

Most of our patients are able to go home and, the next morning, eat a breakfast with sausage, eggs, toast, and fruit. Believe it or not, many patients go to work the next day. The majority of our patients have endured years of dental procedures and dental problems that caused them pain and discomfort, and most are extremely surprised at how comfortable and painless the All-on-4® procedure and recovery are.

Implant Integration
(Osseointegration)

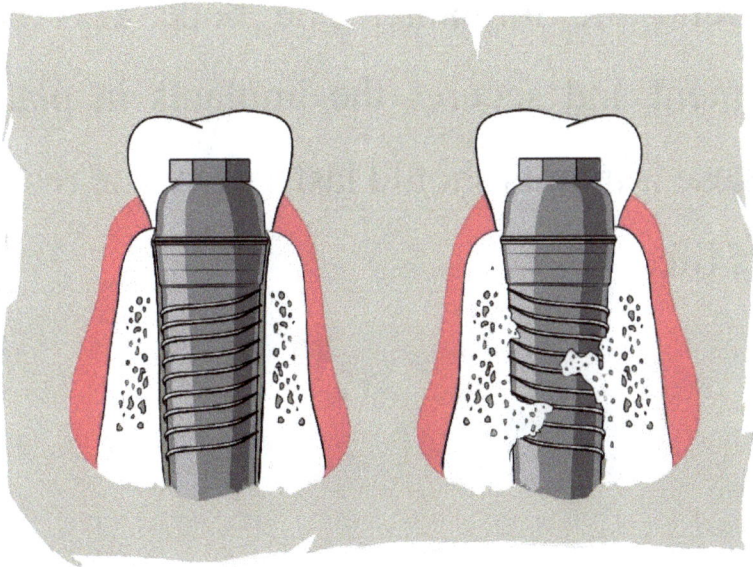

Over the next six months, Trevor's implants go through a process called "osseointegration." This is a fancy word that describes the process of bone growing around the implants. The bone acts like cement and secures the implants in place. These implants should last Trevor the rest of his life.

Trevor's Perfect Smile

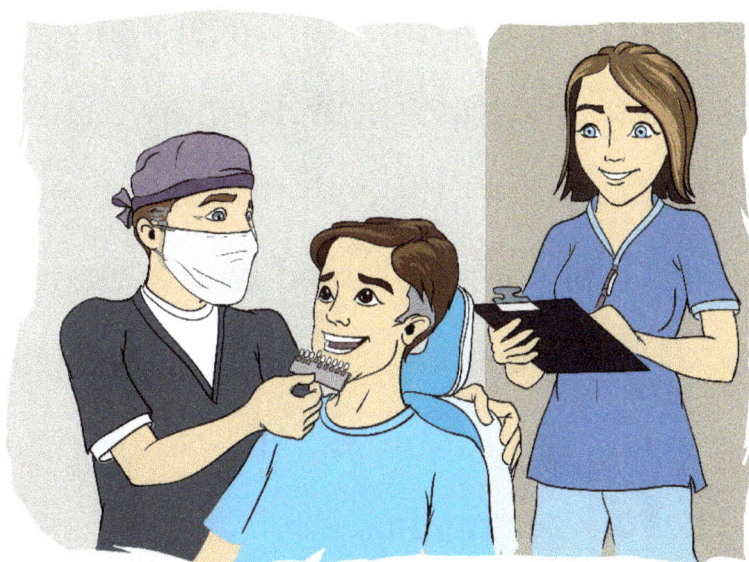

It has been six months and Trevor is ready for his second set of teeth. Even though the first set of teeth are beautiful and strong, they were specifically designed to allow Trevor's gums to heal and the implants to integrate securely. Now, Trevor will get a new set of teeth that are stronger than the first and reinforced with a titanium bar. Everyone notices that Trevor laughs more and smiles more. His smile truly matches his personality.

Trevor's first set of teeth were created to help his implants fully integrate. Now Trevor is getting his final set of teeth.

Trevor got to play a huge role in the way he wanted his second set of teeth to look.

He had the opportunity to work with the lab technician to create his final set. He was given the opportunity to change the color, shape, size, and look of his teeth. Trevor loved his first set of teeth. He said the shape was perfect and natural, but he asked to change the color one shade lighter.

Most people are so happy with the first set that they don't want any physical changes made. The lab technician creates the second set of teeth and infuses a specially milled titanium bar throughout the teeth to make them incredibly strong.

A New Smile, A New Life

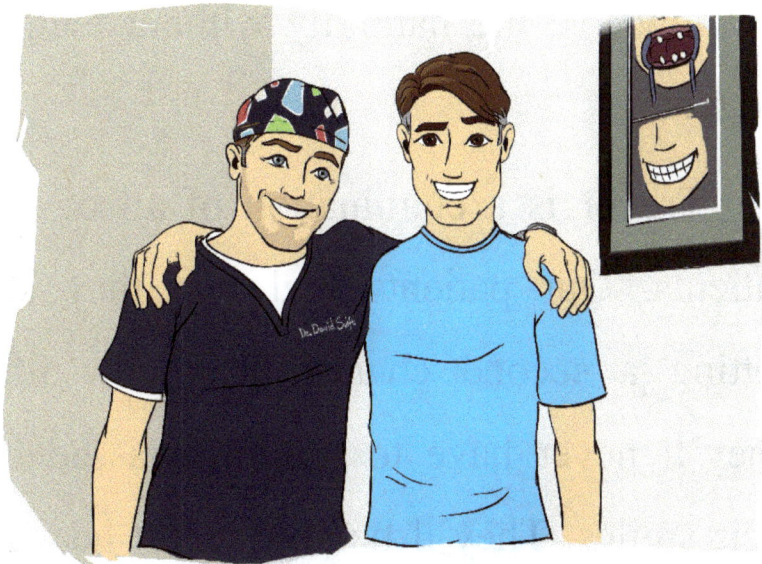

Trevor is amazed by how many people notice his new smile. He says he is overwhelmed by how much happier he feels. He says his life has completely changed – he can now live life naturally without feeling judged.

Trevor is a culmination of all of our patients. Our patients feel that they are getting a second chance at a new life. They'll never have to be embarrassed by their smiles. They'll be able to eat healthy foods again. They will not be overlooked for job opportunities. And they'll never miss another chance to take pictures with their family because they'll no longer feel ashamed of their smile.

To all of the Trevors out there, we can't wait to help you smile again!

For more information on All-On-4® and dental implant books visit our website at www.allon4book.com.

www.ingramcontent.com/pod-product-compliance
Lightning Source LLC
Chambersburg PA
CBHW071520210326
41597CB00018B/2829